...rned on or before
last date below.

D1328875

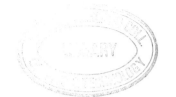

Barbara Woodhouse

on

KEEPING YOUR DOG HEALTHY

RINGPRESS

RINGPRESS

Published by Ringpress Books Ltd,
Spirella House, Bridge Road,
Letchworth, Herts, SG6 4ET

Discounts available for bulk orders
Contact the Special Sales Manager at
the above address. Telephone (0462) 674177

First Published 1992
© 1992 MICHAEL CLAYDON WOODHOUSE

ISBN 0 948955 72 4

Printed and bound in Singapore
by Kyodo Printing Co

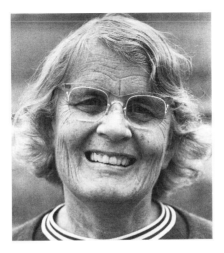

CONTENTS

FOREWORD

By Patrick Woodhouse

My mother was born in Ireland in 1910 at a boys' public school where her father was headmaster. Both her family and the boys at the school had a great many different animals and thus she grew up surrounded by them from a very early age. Dogs and other animals became so much a part of her life that it was obvious from the start that she would have animals around her all her life.

One of my earliest recollections of my mother was that she was always with one or other of her two dogs. In the early Fifties she had a Great Dane which responded so perfectly to her training that it won numerous prizes for obedience work. She realised that she really did have a gift for training dogs and she decided that she must use this gift to help others train their dogs.

She started professionally in 1951 with a dog training club meeting on Croxley Green, just a few yards from our house, which was called Campions. She soon had a class of 25-30 dogs and their owners every Sunday and this led to the founding of four other training clubs, in nearby towns, which were always full of dog owners wishing to learn. Her weekends and evenings were thus spent doing the thing she enjoyed most, the training of dogs.

Her own Great Danes, Juno and Junia, were trained to such a highstandard that they could work in films and on TV programmes by just being shown the action. Then by simply giving them a command or signal, they would act out the part to perfection. Juno, mother's best known Great Dane, became known as " Take 1 Juno" on the sets of the studios where she worked with famous actors like Sir Alec Guinness, Clark Gable, Roger Moore, Eric Morecambe, and many others. Her Great Danes acted in more than eighty TV and movie productions in their careers, and many of the films were produced by my mother and often directed by her as well.

Her career really started to take off when she was invited to do a TV series about dog training for the BBC and the series was to be called: Training Dogs The Woodhouse Way. This series became such a success that it was repeated three times during its first year and led to two more series and a host of appearances on other programmes in which she was interviewed and in which she demonstrated her methods of dog training to TV stars such as Terry Wogan and Michael Parkinson. In the United States the programmes of her dog training became so popular that they are still being shown to this very day. She became known as the "Dog Lady" and her books became some of the best-sellers ever known in America. In 1980 she won the cherished TV award presented by the Pye Corporation as the Female TV Personality Of The Year and went on to win the title of the World's Best Dog Trainer. Since those hectic days she has travelled the world demonstrating her methods to countless dog owners and visiting numerous countries, including the United States of America, Canada, Australia, New Zealand, Singapore and many parts of Europe, before her death in 1988 following a stroke.

I hope that you, the reader, will get a great deal of help from this book and that it will answer all your questions about the difficulties many people experience when training their dogs. I am sure that the sense of achievement you will experience when you have successfully trained your dog to do even the simplest of exercises will give you a sense of oneness with your dog that cannot be bettered by a relationship with any other animal. May I wish you every success with your training and hope that your dog will become, to quote my mother: "A DOG THAT IS A PLEASURE TO ALL AND A NUISANCE TO NO ONE."

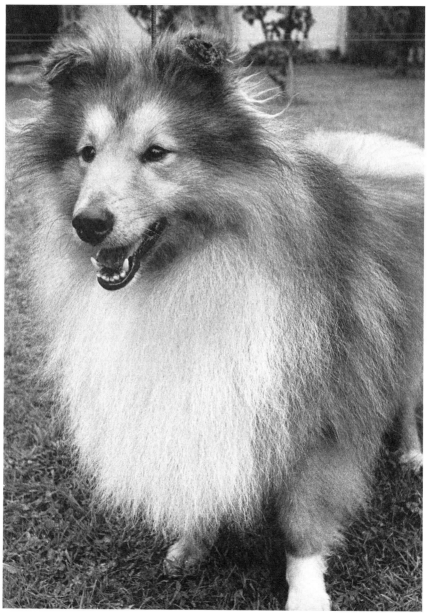

A dog must be kept well-fed and well groomed.

INTRODUCTION

I wonder how many of these ordinary men in the street give much thought to this matter of owning a dog, before they are attracted by a cuddly puppy, with liquid brown eyes, that begs to join you by your fireside? Very few, I am sure. I am therefore going to try to point out the snags that exist and should be considered before any attempt is made to get a dog. First of all, before you buy a dog, decide whether you can afford to give it the home this wonderful friend of man deserves. I don't mean by this that you must be well-off financially to keep a dog. As long as the dog is properly fed, and properly exercised, he is willing to share the humblest abode with his owner. But a dog cannot be kept for nothing. A small dog needs approximately half a pound of meat a day in some form or other, and dog biscuits or brown bread according to its appetite. Therefore I believe that the very lowest sum for which one can keep a dog is about £3 a week. I know that in some households the dog costs nothing, as there are sufficient scraps from the table to give the dog an adequate and balanced diet, but this is the exception rather than the rule. Occasionally the dog becomes ill, and there are charities like the P.D.S.A. who will treat animals free if the owner cannot afford to pay. If every owner depended on this service, the cost of drugs alone would be impossible to meet. So we will conclude that the dog owner should support his own dog.

One must be prepared, too, to spend a small amount on tonics and flea powders, and soaps for washing the dog. No dog that is kept in the house should escape a bath or dry-clean less than once a month. A good many people say to me: "How dogs smell! We would never keep them in the house!" If a dog smells, it is the owner's fault. He wouldn't keep his children unwashed and expect them to remain pleasant companions, yet the dog in some households is expected to keep clean with no help from outside. Have you considered how often the dog dips his mouth into gravy, and milk, into meat or fish, and that some of it is bound to adhere to his lips; yet how many people wash their dog's muzzle occasionally? I clean my dog's muzzle often. But then

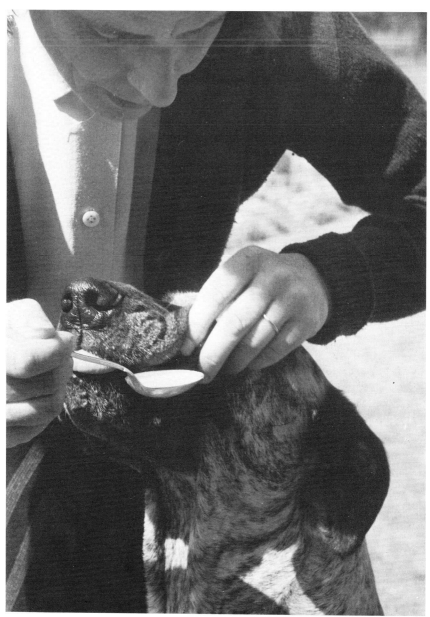

The correct method of giving liquid medicine.

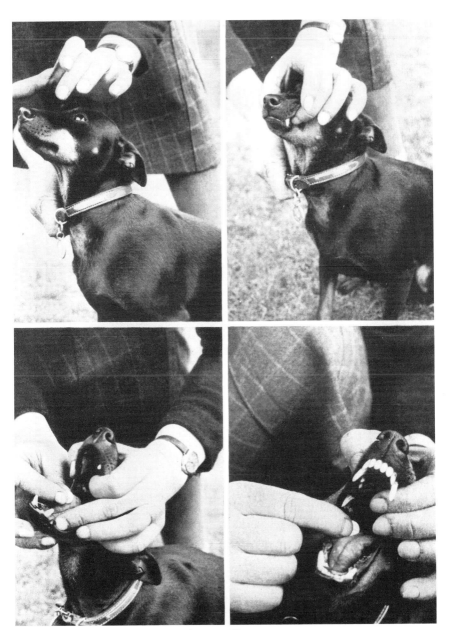

The correct way to give your dog a pill.

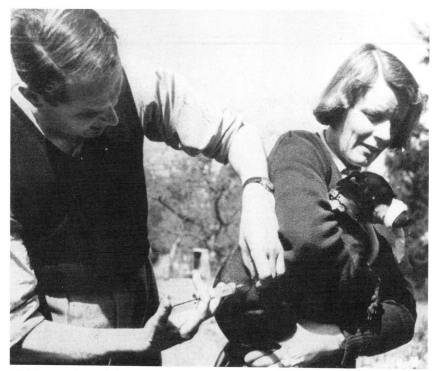

Holding a dog while it is given an injection.

my dog gets a frequent bath with a really easy-lathering soap. The soap not only cleanses her but protects her from any infestation by insects. However clean you keep your dog, if she goes out for walks in the country she is liable to pick up insects. Bathing also helps to get the old coat out, and the rubbing one gives one's dog in lathering the soap acts as a tonic to the skin.

Another frequent complaint is: "My dog's breath smells." Of course it may do, unless you take care to see that your dog eats the right food, that his digestion is in good order, and that his teeth are clean. When one opens some dogs' mouths one is shocked by the state of their teeth. We know such illness as distemper makes the teeth a bad colour, but a lot of this deposit can be removed if, when the dog is ill, his teeth are kept clean with a piece of rag dipped in salt or some toothpaste. At once we hear cries "My dog wouldn't let me open his mouth and do that! He would bite me!" My answer to that is, 'Why haven't you trained your dog better? What happens when you wish to give your dog medicine?' I suppose there is an awful fuss, much growling, and probably spilling of the medicine all over the owner's clothes, with the dog breaking away, and much more friction between dog and owner. I believe that dogs should be trained from early days to sit quietly and have their mouths examined, and their teeth rubbed over; and that if any medicine has to be taken, the dog should be told that he must "come for his medicine". Then, in spite of the fact that the draught is nasty, he must learn to take it without biting or struggling.

With liquid medicine it is easy, as there is a convenient pouch at the side of the dog's mouth; the liquid can be poured into this, and the dog's head tipped gently and down it goes. But with pills it is different. With hungry dogs that bolt their food it is easy to wrap a pill in a piece of meat, and down it all goes without the dog knowing he has taken anything; but with a sick dog who doesn't want to eat anyway, one must know the procedure to follow. I always open the dog's mouth and pop the pill right on the back of the tongue. The dog will move his tongue backwards and forwards in an effort to bring the pill back, but if one tilts the head slightly, down goes the pill. In no circumstances should you push the pill down his throat, or one day you will push it down the windpipe, and choke your dog.

If your vet wishes to give an injection the safest thing to do, if your dog is likely to turn round and bite either you or the vet, is to get a handkerchief and tie it round the dog's mouth. Then you should sit on a sofa or the floor and get the dog to lie down with his head in your lap and your arm over his neck. In this manner the dog cannot see what is going on, and all is over before he has had time to resent it. The mental outlook of the owner towards these operations is very important for the dog

at once picks up the owner's nervous reactions; and people who turn a ghastly white when anything has to be done to their dogs are not the ones to hold them for the vet. The dog senses their nervousness and becomes terrified at once. They should try to get a less squeamish member of the family to help. With a very tiny dog, of course, the previous hints do not apply, since one can mange to hold him for an injection with his head turned away from the vet. I never allow my dogs to be injected on the shoulder. If it has previously hurt, the dog fears that everyone who is going to stroke him may be going to give him another prick. If the injection is made in the loose skin just in front of the flank the dog doesn't seem to mind so much, or to have that same desire to bite when being stroked. Fear is one of the most difficult things to overcome in dogs, and that is why we should do everything in our power to prevent anything happening that is likely to leave fear behind. Never let anyone bend down and stroke your dog when he is asleep. He may wake up in a fright and snap without thinking, then he gets a scolding and your dog has a new problem to overcome.

In the last few years there has been a hate campaign going on about dogs. This has been fuelled by the media, and has led to parents becoming anxious about the risks involved in owning a dog to the health and hygiene of family and home. This is totally exaggerated. There is no risk at all if the necessary precautions are taken to see that a dog is worm-free. Toxocara canis is what the problem is all about, but it can only be passed on to a human if he eats the eggs of the worm that remain in the faeces in the soil. It could therefore be passed to children and could cause blindness in one eye. But the chances of this happening are infinitesimal if sensible precautions are taken and the children made to wash their hands thoroughly before eating. I have been constantly telephoned by people expressing their fears over this, and yet out of a population of fifty million, I could only find eleven cases in a three year period.

It is not possible in a laboratory to tell the difference between Toxocara catis from cats, and Toxocara canis from dogs. Both dogs and cats relieve themselves in the earth and cover it up, so children playing in sandpits could easily come across the faeces of a cat, and could be infected by putting their hands near their mouths. I cannot believe that many children would put faeces-soiled fingers in their mouths. The safeguard is for all dogs and cats to be wormed once or twice a year, and for all strays to be rounded up, then this Toxocara canis scare would completely disappear. The scare has been greatly exaggerated by people who probably hate dogs and spread fear among the dog-owning public out of all proportion to the necessity for the safety of their children's and anybody else's. It has never been a major risk and sensible ownership is the answer.

It is very sad that there are restrictions on where dogs can go these days. In the old days, my animals could go everywhere with me, but now in the interest in hygiene 'No Dogs' read the notices in the shops, and increasingly banning dogs from playing fields and beaches. To my mind, it is much more unhygienic to have people in shops and restaurants sneezing over your cake or pie or touching them with unwashed hands than having a quietly behaved dog in a corner. However, people have reacted strongly to dogs, and I think it is understandable. It is rightfully claimed that you cannot walk on the pavements these days because dog owners do not train their dogs properly. But then, of course, you cannot only blame the dogs but also the indifferent owners for their disregard of the public and cleanliness. If you keep a dog you owe him care and affection. You must look after him in sickness and in health, and you must ensure that he does no harm to anyone. He is your responsibility, and unless you are prepared to take this on, in all its aspects, you should not become a dog owner.

Chapter One

FEEDING

When dogs were still wild animals they chose the food they required in the natural state, and were thus always certain to get what the body required. But nowadays dogs have to rely on the bounty of their owners, and they would receive punishment for helping themselves from the fowl yard when they felt they wanted a chicken. Therefore owners must feed food that is certain to contain all that the dog needs for perfect health. Animals can live for a considerable time without water, but suffer in health as a result of lack of water or water only given spasmodically. Therefore the first rule is to see that there is always a plentiful supply of clean water available day and night for your dog. Without water the dog cannot digest food properly. The nutritional needs of a dog come under two headings, which can best be called the maintenance ration and the production ration. The former represents a bare minimum of feeding which, however, may be quite enough for the old dog lying in the chimney corner all day; the latter simply means

that active, or very active dogs like racing Greyhounds or working hounds, need a good deal of extra food to keep them going.

Before we can examine different methods of feeding dogs we must know a little about the constituents of foods. Carbohydrates are chiefly needed for the production of energy; therefore some kind of biscuits or bread are essential in every dog's diet. Although I have known dogs keep healthy on a diet of meat alone, how long this would last for I don't know. A certain amount of fibre is necessary and helps the passage of waste products in the intestine, though dogs do need less fibre than other domestic animals. Therefore never mash the dog's food too much; this would produce a doughy mass in the intestine and cause trouble. Some hard food is essential for health. Fat provides heat for keeping the dog warm as well as energy, but excessive fat is bad for the dog and tends to give it a bad heart and other troubles. Protein foods like meat and fish are used to build up muscle. If given in excess the

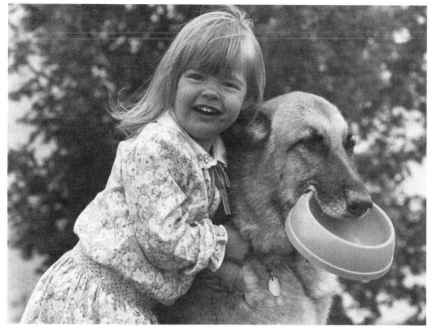

All dogs must receive a well-balanced diet.

strain on the kidneys becomes too much and may cause illness. If too much protein is being decomposed in the intestines it may cause diarrhoea. Thus it will be seen that in every case feeding must be balanced for the good health of the dog.

Minerals are absolutely essential for the well-being of the dog. They are required for bone formation in the growing animal and for the healthy state of the blood and tissues. Normally a well-balanced diet will contain enough minerals for all the dog's needs, but if the dog doesn't receive enough minerals from his food the body draws on the bones and tissues. Lack of minerals causes rickets, and also (coupled with lack of vitamins A and D) causes slow recovery after a feverish illness. It causes

eczema, and some people even hold it responsible for cases of hysteria. Remember that puppies draw their mineral needs from their dam, so it is especially necessary to provide calcium and phosphorus, in particular, for the use of the dam's body. Calcium is present in milk and bones or can be given by mouth in proprietary products. Eclampsia in a bitch (a disease which often occurs some days after whelping) is caused by lack of calcium. This is a very dangerous trouble and can cause death if the lack of calcium is not made good by injection. The animal becomes highly excitable and may collapse; veterinary aid must be sought quickly. Mineral deficiency should be suspected in the following cases: if the legs of growing puppies are not straight, and bulge at the joints; if their coats are not shiny, and if they are always scratching, in spite of the fact that they have no infestation by insects. There are a vast number of products on the market which provide minerals and vitamins and everything else necessary for the dog's health, and nowadays there is ample knowledge of the uses of minerals in the nutrition of the dog.

Dogs require concentrated food; they are not like cows who have four stomachs and can regurgitate and chew again what they have eaten. A dog has only one stomach which must not be abused. Half their diet should be of meat, with occasional changes to fish. When puppies are being reared remember bitches' milk is far richer than cows' milk, and more closely resembles the milk of goats (which many breeders keep for this reason). Cows' milk can be made more like bitches' milk by gently simmering it and getting rid of some of the water.

Normally dogs need only two meals a day, at midday and at night. The biggest meal should always be at night when the dog has time to sleep and digest his food. Hounds are seldom fed daily. They get enormous meals three times a week and seem to keep extremely fit on this diet, but it would not suit the ordinary dog owner to feed her dog in this way, although it is quite a well-known custom to starve a dog one day a week. This I have never done, nor would I like to start it. I think regular mealtimes are most important in the life of a healthy dog. The saliva begins to flow at the usual time for a meal and the digestive juices, if not employed, may in my opinion cause digestive upsets. If a dog doesn't get his expected meal you are letting him down and his faith in you cannot be as strong as it should be. I never let a dog down in any way if I can help it.

FEEDING PUPPIES

There are few hard and fast rules about feeding dogs. Like babies, puppies vary enormously in what they like and what is good for them and their appetites vary even within the same litter. When the puppy first comes into your home at about eight to ten weeks or even earlier, he must be fed four or five times a day according to his appetite. Small meals, easily digested, should be the rule. The diet should include minced raw beef, milk, brown bread or puppy meal and a plentiful supply of clean water. Additional vitamins should be added to the diet to ensure freedom from rickets; cod-liver oil or proprietary brands of vitamins A, D and also B are the most important for health and growth.

It is impossible to lay down exact amounts for each puppy, but in the main they should have two meat meals a day and two milk ones. Reduce this number to two a day gradually, so that at about six to eight months the puppy has one or two meals a day only. To ensure sleep at night give the biggest meal last. Nowadays there are so many proprietary brands of food available, each with full instructions enclosed, that no one, however lacking in knowledge, need feed their dog wrongly. However, what will make one puppy thrive will upset another. I have often found that it is necessary to change a puppy's brand of food, not because there is anything wrong with that particular brand, but because it just doesn't suit that particular animal.

Vegetables are not, as many people believe, a necessity. Some puppies love them, and they certainly do no harm, but they do not form part of a dog's natural diet. Bones are not really good for dogs – they not only cause constipation but can so easily splinter and lead to internal injury – but puppies do like a big shin-bone to grind their teeth on. Meat for puppies should of course be minced, and the occasional addition of such things as egg or liver to the diet can do nothing but good. Chocolates, sweets, and highly seasoned foods are good for neither puppies nor fully-grown dogs, and begging for scraps from the human's table must be firmly discouraged. Let the puppies be fed at their own mealtimes only, and stick to these times religiously.

GENERAL GUIDE FOR FEEDING MEDIUM-SIZED DOGS WEIGHING FROM 20-30LBS WHEN ADULT.

(Smaller or larger breeds in proportion)

EIGHT TO TWELVE WEEKS

7.30am: Drink of warm cow's milk.

9.30am: 11/2 oz of fresh or tinned meat and half a teacupful of puppy meal or two slices of brown bread, soaked in meat stock.

3pm: Drink of milk with brown bread or a puppy biscuit.

6pm: 11/2 oz minced beef cooked or raw or tinned meat with cornflakes or half a cupful of soaked puppy meal.

10.pm: Drink of warm milk.

TWELVE WEEKS TO SIX MONTHS

7.30am: Drink of cow's milk, two toasted slices of brown bread with butter or a few ovals or puppy meal.

12 noon: 2-4oz tinned meat or minced cooked beef or fish (Coley).

6.pm: 2-4oz fresh or tinned meat mixed with dry brown bread on half a cup of puppy meal soaked beforehand. A drink of milk.

SIX MONTHS ONWARDS

As a dog reaches six months and over, the feeds are gradually reduced to two a day, 1/2lb of beef or one small tin of dog meat and about a teacupful of biscuit meal and a drink of milk should keep a dog healthy, providing vitamins are added to the diet in some form.

GRASS-EATING

This is purely and simply the dog's method of making himself sick and relieving some indisposition of the digestion. Bilious dogs do it to get rid of the excessive bile built up in the stomach and after being sick will very often feel quite all right and be ready for a meal. I have heard it said that dogs left to wander in the countryside eat all sorts of greenstuffs which is taken to mean that they lack vegetables in their diet. I have never had this happen with my own dogs or the people's dogs I have boarded, so I am inclined to think that a dog properly fed does not indulge in this habit.

Chapter Two

HOUSING

I think all dogs become much nicer dogs when living in close contact with their owners, so the ideal situation is for all owners to keep their dogs in their homes with them, with the addition of a wire indoor kennel. This is very useful when you are house training, and it gives the dog a place where he can rest in peace, out of harm's way. If you decide to keep your dog in the house, let him get used to sleeping in the kitchen. where there is a tiled or linoleum floor. If he does this, and then owing to tummy trouble, there is an accident, you will not feel like murder. A house trained dog should never be scolded for an accident he could not help because there was nobody there to let him out.

There are all manner of beds, baskets and beanbags currently on the market for dogs, and your choice must be guided by personal preference and the money you want to spend. However, I think the round-shaped baskets for dogs are an abomination. They make the dog sleep in a curled up position instead of stretched out, which is natural and more restful for the dog. If you do not want to go to the expense of buying a dog bed, it is a perfectly simple matter to make a bed at home, with three sides of wood, and the bottom made either of wood or webbing like a sofa. Bedclothes should consist of padded bedding or the dog's folded blanket. Every dog should have two blankets, which must be laundered fairly frequently to keep the bed clean and sweet-smelling. This type of bed is suitable for medium-sized terriers and bigger dogs, but I think tiny mites prefer an indoor kennel. If you are rich you can buy the most beautifully made ones, lined with silk; but you can also make one at home out of a wooden box in exactly the same manner as a rabbit hutch.

OUTSIDE KENNELS

If you are a breeder with a large number of dogs, obviously you must keep your dogs in kennels. But this problem of the owner who has a job and is away for long periods of each day, is always a difficult one. It seems unfair to a dog lover to deny him or her the love and companionship of a dog under these

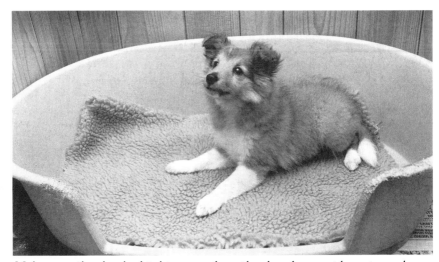

Make sure the dog bed is big enough so the dog does not have to curl up.

circumstances. The life of an only dog is something like that of an only child, and I always ask the future owner if it would not be possible to keep two dogs as companions for each other. I feel a kennel where the dogs could play together would be ideal. If, on the other hand, it is only possible to have one dog and the dog is kept in the house, the problem arises of what happens if the poor dog has a tummy upset and cannot get out to relieve himself. A house trained dog would suffer tortures of remorse if this happened. If, on the other hand, this happened to a kennel dog the run would be used, and no harm done.

I think the construction of the kennel matters a lot. The most perfect range of kennels I ever saw was at the Guide Dogs For The Blind Association. Two dogs shared each kennel, where this was possible, and they had a raised bench to sleep on. Ventilation was provided by grating as well as a door and window, and they had a lovely concrete run. The doors were sheet-metal lined to save them from being gnawed. This kind of thing is obviously beyond the average owner's pocket, but a vast number of manufactures of kennels do produce a great variety of types. Of course, kennel accom-modation depends on the breed of dog you want. A German Shepherd, for example, has a weather-proof coat and can stand cold weather as long as he is dry and out of draughts, whereas a short-coated dog would suffer it not kept much warmer.

Naturally, guard duties are better performed by a dog kept indoors, and few burglars will burgle a house if they know a large or medium-sized dog is kept there. However, if the owner of a dog has to be away most of the day, the dog must have an outside kennel and be exercised before the owner leaves in the morning and after he comes home at night. Some people think such an

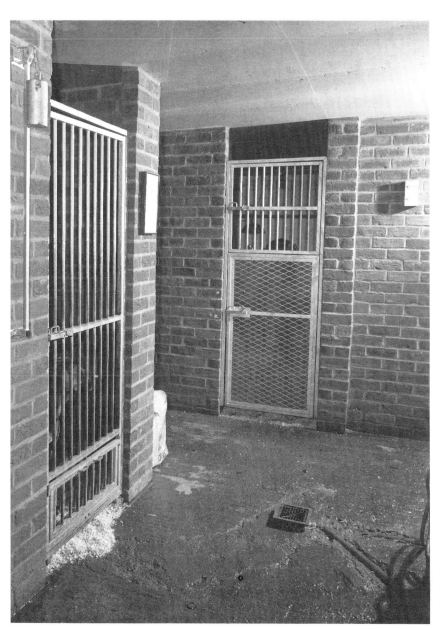

Part of a brick-built kennel block

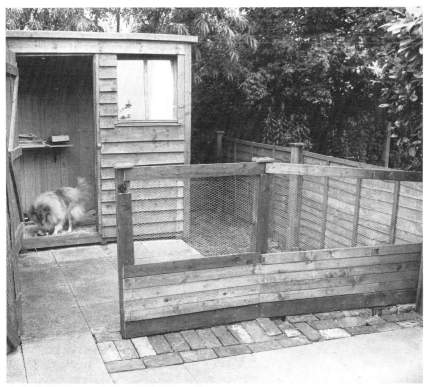

A different type of outside kennel.

arrangement is cruel, but dogs soon get accustomed to routine and hundreds of show dogs live this life. The dog should come into its own at weekends if it can be with the owner most of the day, especially if it is allowed in the house.

BOARDING KENNELS

If you cannot take your dog on holiday he must, of course, be boarded, though I hope this is not being done because the dog is not well-behaved enough to

be taken with you. If that is the case do start training it to lie down and stay down alone each day, as many hotels allow well-behaved dogs in their owners' bedrooms. However, if you are going abroad you must of course find a suitable holiday home for him. Many of the animal welfare societies have lists of approved kennels. If you can find someone who has boarded their dog out in satisfactory kennels, a personal knowledge of these holiday homes is by far the best recommendation.

Chapter Three

GENERAL CARE

EXERCISE

A lot of nonsense is talked about exercising dogs. Most people are exercising themselves more than the dog when they stroll round the town shop-gazing, or walk twice round the block at night. If you cannot give your dog walks he can be let out to amuse himself in the garden if the weather is fine. A lot of people, many of them elderly folk, who should be looking after their own health, make martyrs of themselves exercising dogs in all weathers. Do the best you can for your pet and he will not hold it against you that he has missed the smells of the countryside. Dogs soon accustom themselves to a certain routine when they know no other. Exercise has two sides to it. There is that essential amount of movement necessary to keep the dog in good health, and that extra exercise that gives the dog and possibly the owner pleasure, but which is not a necessity. The first must be given, the second need not. A dog picks up his owner's moods and in some cases never asks for a walk if he thinks his owner is too worried or busy to come out, yet the slightest sign of a changed mood on the owner's part and the dog is waiting and ready to have fun. That is the joy of owning an intelligent dog.

I would, however, stress to all owners that some dogs need masses of exercise to keep them happy and free from annoying habits and vices. Some dogs need to follow a master or mistress on foot or on horseback for miles each day (or even follow a car if properly trained to stay on the grass verge). Some dogs are never still, they are always begging to be taken out. These are tiresome dogs to own if you are a busy person, yet there is no particular breed of which one can say firmly that they need tons of exercise. I have known Boxers who were never still, and I know Boxers who can hardly be dragged out for a walk. It is all according to the individual make-up of particular dogs. It also depends on your initial training when the dog first comes into your home. You may at first be so thrilled with the fact that you own a dog that you take him out for long walks daily. The dog loves this and begins to know the routine. As the

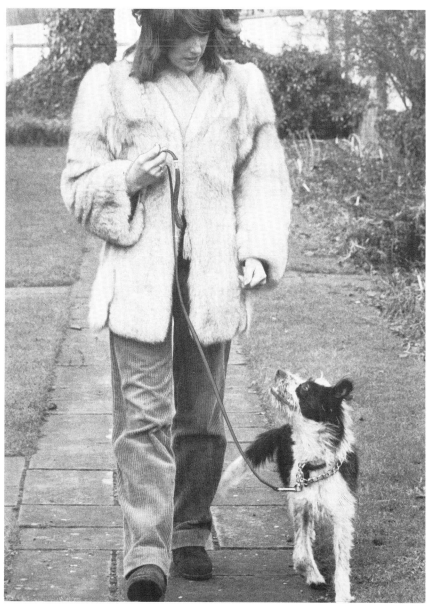

Dogs are creatures of habit, so adopt an exercise routine that you know you can keep to.

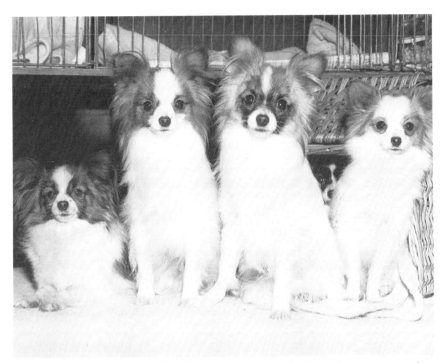

A small breed such as a Papillon does not need a lot of exercise, and is suitable for the elderly or infirm owner.

owner's new enthusiasm wears thin the dog gets less and less exercise and thereby hangs a tale, for this is what makes a dog tear things up and become a problem to handle. They are creatures of routine, so start as you really mean to go on, and don't get carried away in the beginning by enthusiasm you cannot hope to maintain.

If you are elderly or suffer from some infirmity, this does not mean that you cannot own a dog. But I do think that you should be most careful in the type of dog you choose if you have an infirmity. I think you should buy a tiny toy dog and would suggest an older dog rather than a puppy. If possible choose one that might be likely to want to chase a ball for exercise. Yorkshire Terriers are very sporting and will retrieve a ball for as long as you like to throw one. Neither Pomeranians nor Papillons need much exercise.

GROOMING

Grooming aids circulation and the casting of the old coat; it helps the skin to breathe by friction and is excellent for promoting health in dogs. Most dogs need some grooming, however perfunctory. Some dogs need a tremendous amount of care of the coat, and if you want a dog in tip-top

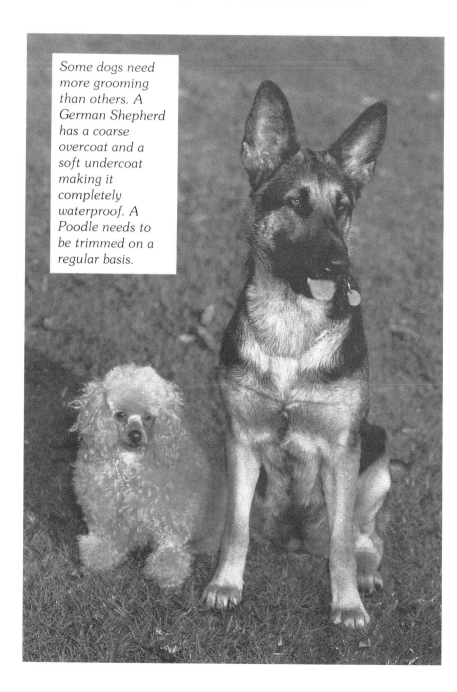

Some dogs need more grooming than others. A German Shepherd has a coarse overcoat and a soft undercoat making it completely waterproof. A Poodle needs to be trimmed on a regular basis.

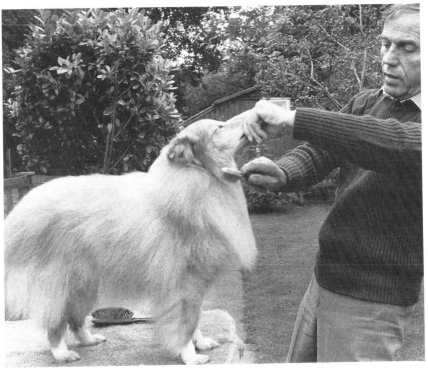

A long-coated breed such as a Shetland Sheepdog should be brushed and combed on a daily basis.

condition, groom him even if it is only once a week. A glove brush is the most suitable for short-coated dogs, a wire brush and comb for long-haired dogs. Some people carry out their own stripping; a stripping comb specially made for the job with one sharp edge can be used. Some dogs are far more sensitive than others, so when you groom your dog be careful not to be rough or you will make him bad-tempered. I have a lot of pupils in my training schools who come because they bite their owners when groomed. Groom firmly but gently – remember how it hurts you to have your hair

pulled! On the other hand you must be firm about carrying out grooming irrespective of the dog's wishes; once he learns that you stop grooming him when he bites, the seed is well and truly sown.

There are two types of hair in most dogs' coats, the overlength hair which is the coarse, long hair, and the undercoat which is the soft hair underneath. In dogs like German Shepherds this makes the coat completely waterproof. In trimming a dog it is the long overlength hairs which should be plucked out, leaving the softer undercoat intact. That is why just clipping instead of plucking

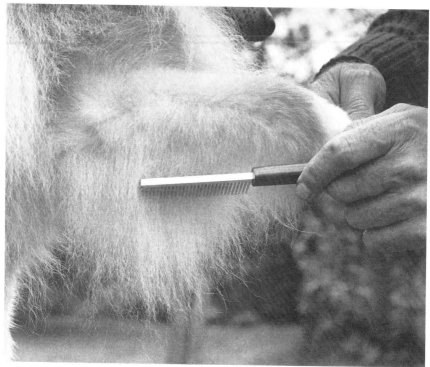

Particular attention should be paid to the leg fringes where the hair can become matted.

the coat out is not so good for the dog as correct stripping, which gets rid of the loose old hair. Terriers need trimming three or four times a year, and unless you are very good at it I think it is better to take the dog to a professional stripper. A terrier badly done looks awful, and the same applies to Poodles and Cocker Spaniels. The cost, we know, adds up, but if money is very tight I do not imagine you would buy a dog that needed a lot of beauty attention.

BATHING

There is no hard and fast rule as to how often to bath a dog. I think a good bath once a month with a good dog soap helps circulation and aids casting out of the old coat, but if your dog seems perfectly healthy-coated and clean, there is no need to worry. However, if your dog smells or is scratching, or losing his coat excessively, I should bath him. If his coat is clean and shiny and you groom him regularly, I think he shouldn't be bathed more than once every three months. Bathing softens the coat, and takes away natural oil, although the friction from rubbing the dog dry and the getting out of the old coat more than makes up for these

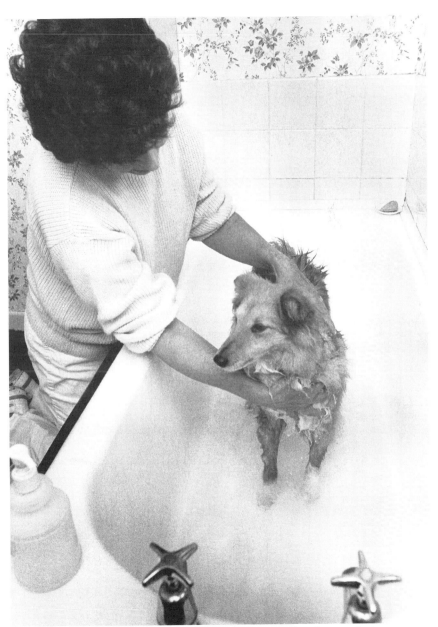

A bath keeps a dog clean and sweet-smelling and aids circulation.

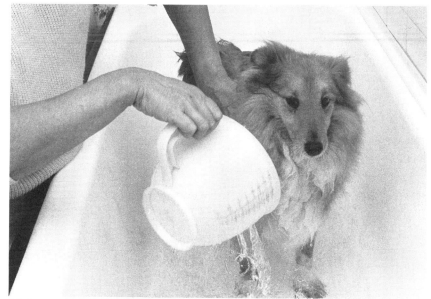

Make sure all the shampoo is rinsed out.

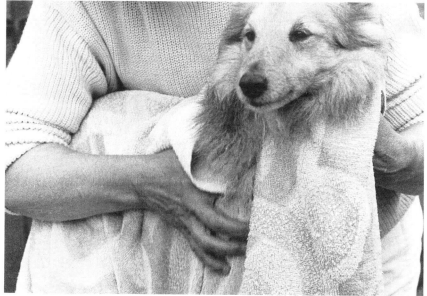

After a bath the dog will need to be dried thoroughly.

things. Always use a good dog soap, there are many brands, and the result should be a nice sweet-smelling clean dog.

Bathing in the sea is not good for dogs' coats and often leads to eczema. Let him bathe if he wishes, but pop him into the bath afterwards and rinse the salt out with warm water before drying him. Otherwise the salt leaves a deposit in the coat which eventually leads to scratching. The long-coated breeds suffer from this more than the short-coated ones. If you want proof that sea water is bad for hair go to the sea and see what a state your own hair is in after a few days of the briny.

EARS

Many people poke their dogs' ears with cotton buds in the mistaken idea that the inner ear must be cleaned regularly. This is wrong. It is far safer to inject a little warm oil into the ear, or some ear-drops. Then the wax will be lubricated and will come out when the ear is shaken by the dog. The outer ear should always be kept clean from the brown discharge, which denotes ear trouble, but usually an infective, not a parasitic one. Antibiotic ear-drops soon clear this up. As soon as the dog holds his head on one side, or shakes it, or scratches it, get expert advice.

Never allow water or soap to enter the inner ear; plug the ear with cotton wool before treating the outer flap. Sometimes the hair gets matted in breeds like Spaniels, and it must then be cut off or a weeping eczema starts. Calamine lotion and ear-drops usually clear up this trouble once air has been allowed to enter the ear. There is no

disease called 'canker' – this is only a name that covers a multitude of troubles, coined for lay use. Find out the specific cause and treat accordingly.

NAIL CLIIPPING

Most dogs who get regular road exercise need little attention to their nails, but dogs whose exercise is mostly taken on grass do need them cutting about once a month. This cutting should either be done by an expert or at home with proper nail-clippers. It should never be attempted with scissors. The nail might break and cause severe pain to the dog.

The length of nail varies considerably according to the breed and also between dogs of a particular breed. I owned a Miniature Black-and-Tan Terrier that had never been able to have her nails cut. I only tried once and hurt the quick, in spite of the fact that the nail looked as if it needed cutting. These nails never grew any longer in five years, yet her companion, my Great Dane Juno, had her nails cut every three weeks. They both had the same amount of exercise.

When the nails are white the quick can be easily seen and the nail can be then cut to about one-sixth of an inch off the quick. If the dog flinches don't cut it so short. If a dog should break or split a nail, wrap the nail round with Elastoplast strapping and it will soon be all right again.

DEW CLAWS

In my opinion dew-claws should be removed when a puppy is a few days old for its health and safety, and the

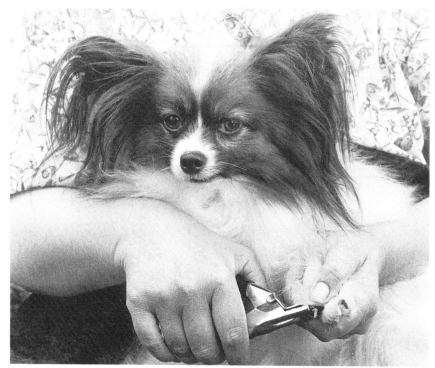

Nails should be trimmed if they grow too long – guillotine nail-clippers are the easiest to use.

safety of its owner. Dew-claws can grow inwards and cause the dog intense pain, or they can tear clothes as the dog jumps up. They are of no practical use to the dog. Some breeds, however, like Pyrenean Mountain Dogs have double dew-claws, which are part and parcel of the Breed Standard, and must be kept intact – why, I utterly fail to understand. But then there is a lot in the doggy world I fail to understand! The removal of dew-claws can be done very easily with a sharp pair of surgical scissors curved outwards. The claws are cut off as near the leg as is practical without injuring the skin. Friar's Balsam is applied to the incision; nothing more need be done. In my opinion it is better to remove both front and back dew-claws, as I have seen dogs with nasty leg wounds where the dew-claws have caught in something and torn away.

TEETH

Puppies do not have teeth when they are born, but round about the eighteenth day the first ones should pierce the gums. This rate varies according to the breed of dog; some get their teeth out a little later. The first teeth are called milk teeth and number twenty-eight. They are pointed and smaller than the permanent teeth of which there are normally forty-two (but occasionally forty-four in large breeds). By about the fifth week the puppies have a complete set. Owing to the rather softer make-up of these milk teeth they wear more easily than the permanent ones and the points of the incisors and tusks are often worn off.

Occasionally the milk teeth are not cast before the permanent ones make their appearance, and it is then necessary to take the offending milk teeth out. Usually, however, if the puppies are given hard biscuits, or large bones that can't splinter their teeth, they will come out by themselves. Dentition is completed round about the fourth month in big breeds and rather later in smaller breeds. Teething time can be a troublesome one, when puppies have been known to get eczema or convulsions. The puppy should be wormed at round about four months, as it is often the worms that are causing the convulsions rather than teething. Remember also that milk is essential in the diet of all young dogs. Dogs fed almost entirely on soft foods suffer with tartar much more than dogs that are given something hard to masticate. Scraping the tartar off the dog's teeth is done by experts and should be done if tartar is present in quantity, as otherwise the gum will be affected and an unhealthy state of the mouth will develop. The dog will get bad breath, and eventually loss of teeth and digestive upsets may follow.

The care of the teeth, in fact, is most important. I clean my dogs' teeth with salt on a damp rag, but any tooth powder made for human use will serve, or any of the manufactured toothpastes made specially for dogs. Dogs should be trained from an early age to have their mouths examined and handled. Incidentally it takes an expert to judge the dog's age by its teeth after dentition is complete; as the years pass the age can only be roughly estimated by the yellow state of the teeth and the presence of tartar. If a dog is allowed to chew on a marrow bone this will help to keep his teeth clean.

BAD ODOURS

The dog that smells, or has bad breath is an anti-social creature, and it is the responsibility of the owner to ensure that the dog is kept clean and sweet-smelling. Tooth decay and the accumulation of tartar can be a cause of bad breath, and therefore teeth should be checked regularly. You should also wash your dog's mouth occasionally. Think of all the food, and dirty things as well, that he touches with his lips. The liquid from over-full anal glands makes a dog smell terribly. If this is the cause get them squeezed by a vet. Flatulence is caused by a too fatty diet; correct this and one source of doggy odours is dispelled. Urine from a male dog makes more of a smell than that from a bitch; wash the dog in a good dog-soap and that particular smell will go. Vitamin A in large doses for a few weeks helps digestion and reduces the risk of bowel flatulence. Discharge of any sort from the vagina of a bitch smells horrid and needs instant attention. It might be the start of Pyometra or inflammation in the womb. Certain skin diseases like mange have a horrible smell. Examine the dog for any bare patches if this is found to be the cause.

THE ELDERLY DOG

The lifespan of a dog depends on so many things: the home the dog lives in, whether he is fed on a sensible diet, given proper exercise, and kept reasonably slim. It also depends on the size of the dog. Small dogs live longer than large breeds. For example a Great Dane's life is not usually much longer than ten or eleven years, whereas I have known a Manchester Terrier that was eighteen years old. My neighbours' Fox Terrier is already thirteen, but full of beans. Normally, though, I think that if a dog reaches the age of twelve it has nearly had its span of life.

Remember dogs need less exercise as they get older, and much less food. They sleep for long periods at a time, and the owner should no longer force the dog to go for long walks when he seems disinclined to do so. With bitches watch carefully the heat period and make sure they have no evil-smelling discharge. Pyometra is very common in aged bitches and can be fatal. Pyometra is an inflammation of the womb, and pus gets locked up inside and causes acute infection if not dealt with either by antibiotics, or in many cases that operation for the removal of the female organs which is known as partial or complete hysterectomy according to the organs removed. As a precaution I always put my own bitch on antibiotics for three days after her heat is finished. Before I did this she was always dull and listless although nothing like an emergency flared up. Now she returns to her old self very quickly. Many people ask me when bitches stop coming on heat. The answer is that they don't have a menopause as we know it,

and heat continues as long as the bitch lives. That does not, of course, mean they are always capable of breeding; very often they refuse to produce puppies some years before they are really old. One should watch for blindness and deafness in old dogs. I know several people who keep dogs whose sight has almost entirely gone. Whether this is cruelty or kindness is a point for discussion but I think it is cruel. I think in most cases the owner lacks the courage to put the pet to sleep. Deafness, however, is not in my opinion in the same category because I have trained a few dogs deaf from birth and found them quite trainable and able to enjoy life like normal dogs. Some dogs get incontinent and get sore from urine perpetually dripping over their hindquarters. This is unpleasant for both owner and dog, and, after taking professional advice as to whether any treatment will cure this trouble and finding the answer to be in the negative, I think the animal should be put to sleep. Such dogs cannot sleep in the house without constant change of bedding and even then the smell is horrid. They drink excessive amounts of water which usually also denotes kidney failure, and altogether the dog's life cannot be a very happy one. When the time comes to make the decision to end a dog's life, I suggest you ask your vet to give you some sleeping tablets that you can put into your's dog's food. The dog will naturally go to sleep in his own home, and the vet can then be called to inject him with a fatal dose. The dog will know nothing and feel nothing. You owe this to a faithful friend, so do not shirk your duty, however terrible for you.

Chapter Four

BREEDING

The majority of the dog-owning public do not want to become involved in breeding a litter. Owners of bitches do not want to go to the trouble and expense of rearing a litter, and then having to find good homes for the resulting puppies. Owners of dogs do not want their pet to start mating bitches, and becoming more like a stud dog than a member of the family. There still goes around the old wives' tale that if you don't breed with a bitch she will get ill and her uterus will get diseased. This is nonsense; Pyometra (pus in the womb) happens just as often in bitches that have had puppies as with those that have not, probably more.

The other fallacy is that to breed with a bitch stops her having false pregnancies or pseudo-pregnancies as they are called. This is not so. I once owned a bitch that had had six litters, and she had the most realistic false pregnancies so that I really began to wonder whether she had somehow got away and got mated. She had every symptom of pregnancy, and all the drugs that the vet prescribed did no good at all. She tore up my sofa every time and anything else she could get hold of; this was her pathetic method of making a nest. Never breed unless you want to do so for pleasure or profit. If you do not fall into either of these categories – and the majority of dog owners do not – your aim is to prevent your dog or bitch from breeding. I will therefore deal with this subject first, before going into the practical details of breeding a litter.

BITCHES ON HEAT

Nowadays the use of chlorophyll in large doses has been found to be extremely effective in preventing male dogs from picking up the strong scent emitted by a bitch on heat, and I have also proved with my own bitches that by commencing dosing according to the directions with Amplex brand of chlorophyll they can be taken out comfortably without being molested by dogs. Some people even take them to shows – with the exception of obedience shows which are barred to bitches on heat by Kennel Club rules – and the dogs completely ignore the

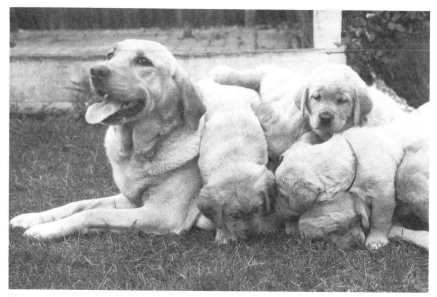

Puppies are always appealing, but do not be tempted to breed with your bitch unless you have thought about all the implications.

bitches' presence.

I have run residential dog training courses at my home with male dogs in the house and my own two bitches on heat, and no male dog fussed or made any attempt to get near my bitches when they were dosed as mentioned. But I do think one is taking an unnecessary risk if one does not closely confine the bitches for the last five days of the heat period, owing to the fact that the bitches themselves are extremely provocative towards any dog at this vital stage and do everything in their power to attract the male dog.

The quantity of chlorophyll to be given depends entirely on the size and weight of the dog. Directions are enclosed and the owner of each dog must work out what that particular dog needs. The substance is quite harmless,

so no one need be frightened of giving an overdose. It is always helpful to wash the bitch's vulva two or three times a day with chlorophyll dissolved in spirit. If possible exercise her away from your own premises. I used to take my bitches in the car some distance away before letting them run, thus if there were any scent to be picked up it would not lead the male dogs to my house.

Most people want to know when to start dosing their bitches with chlorophyll. The answer is as soon as you notice the swelling of the bitch's vulva and the discharge of blood from the genital passage. The period of heat varies vastly in bitches but nine to fifteen days is about average. Some bitches only come on heat once a year, some as many as four times a year. The greatest number do so twice a year. The bitch is ready for mating as the discharge lessens and she stands with her tail turned sideways. This is the time when, whether using chlorophyll or not, I recommend careful isolation from any male dog for nineteen days. Should the 'on heat' bitch escape and be accidentally mated, heat can be brought on again by Stilboestrol given by the vet and the pregnancy terminated. This however must be done quickly. The old idea that if a bitch escapes and gets mated by a mongrel she will for ever be ruined is rubbish. Telegony, as it is called, has many followers, but scientifically it is nonsense. What is possible, however, is for a bitch to have pure-bred puppies and mongrels in the same litter, for a bitch will mate several times with different dogs and each mating can produce puppies. The pure-bred ones will be pure-bred and not in any way tainted for future use in the breed, and the mongrels will be forever crossbreds. That is how this telegony idea has grown up. Naturally the person who has been careless enough to let a valuable bitch out whilst on heat and get mated is not going to admit it.

CASTRATION

Some males make very nice pets, and their owners have no problems with them either chasing after bitches on heat, or becoming over-sexed and indulging in anti-social behaviour such as mounting legs or cushions, or lifting their leg at every lampost. However, in my opinion, the best thing to do if the dog is not wanted for breeding or showing is to get the vet to castrate him. I know of no ill effects after this operation, and I cannot imagine why

more dogs are not operated on. They do not lose their character, nor do they become fat, with judicious feeding. They are gay, happy dogs and much nicer to own. That is more than I can say for bitches that have been spayed (had their ovaries removed). They become dull, lazy and run to fat very easily as they get older.

A veterinary surgeon writes: "This operation is comparatively simple and consists of the surgical removal of both testicles. This, of course, necessitates a general anaesthetic, but with modern methods of anaesthesia and a healthy animal, that presents very little risk. Each testicle is then removed by making an incision in the scrotal sac, ligating the spermatic cord and excising the organ. The wound is left to drain and is not sutured, healing very rapidly, being complete in seven days. Within a fortnight the adult animal is completely recovered, and is ready to resume training.

"The result of this operation becomes apparent during the ensuing months. The animal no longer shows any sexual excitement in the presence of other dogs or bitches, becomes more amenable, and responds more readily to training, without losing any of his joie de vivre. Of course, the loss of his sexual interest results in a greater interest in food and comfort. The animal is more eager for his meals and readily clears up much more than he actually requires.

Owners should not succumb to the temptation of over feeding, as there is a tendency for the animal to put on weight. Excessive weight is very hard to reduce once it has been allowed to develop.

MONORCHIDS AND CRYPTORCHIDS

These terms are used for male dogs whose testicles have not descended normally. Monorchid means that only one testicle has descended into the scrotum, and cryptorchid means neither testicle has descended. A monorchid can still beget puppies, but both defects, in my opinion, make the dog a bad one for it may have a very uncertain temperament. I find them extremely difficult to train, and recommend castration. This is also more difficult than usual to do as the undescended testicle has to be found before the operation of castration can be performed. Inexperienced dog buyers may buy one of these and get badly bitten as they are usually appalling fighters as well. In fact, I can see nothing to recommend keeping one.

PRINCIPLES OF BREEDING

If you are going to take up dog breeding seriously you must read books specially written on the subject; you must attend shows, and study heredity, breeding for certain qualities, line-breeding and in-breeding. First of all you must realise what you are aiming at. People imagine that if they buy a bitch with 'Champion' written in red ink all over her pedigree they are certain to have a perfect dam to start breeding with. All they have to do is find the equally marvellous sire with red ink 'Champion' all over his pedigree, and the resulting litter will be perfect. How wrong they are! To get the perfect puppy, let alone the perfect litter, is something that takes experienced breeders often a lifetime of trial and error, and will hardly ever be achieved at the first attempt.

We know the old saying 'like begets like' but what we may not know is what characteristics past generations have passed on to dam and sire. Such characteristics may not be discernible in the parents-to-be, yet a mating could produce something vastly different to what we expected. Only by having litters can one prove what that particular mating will produce. Always remember that dam and sire exert equal influence on the litter, and it may therefore be unfair to blame the sire for the faults of the offspring. Choose your bitch just as carefully as you choose your sire, and remember temperament. This is most important. For however good the puppies, if they are nervous or fierce they will not be welcomed either as pets or for show purposes. Both sides should be chosen for the greatest number of desirable qualities in each, and for their ability to stamp these qualities on their offspring. Therefore, if possible, see stock that the sire has fathered and note any good or bad points. For the mating together of two animals with the same good or bad points tends to fix these points and, in the case of the bad ones, they are almost sure to be passed on by the offspring when they breed in turn.

This brings me to in-breeding which is of course the mating together of closely related dogs, and is done in the hope of stamping certain good qualities in those dogs on their offspring. 'Line-breeding' is simply choosing dogs from the same line of descent to be mated together with the same object of accumulating blood on both sides that you particularly like in your breed of dog. There is much that can be written about both methods, but the most dangerous to dabble in is in-breeding as the mated dogs have practically the same ancestors and you may therefore again find that not only have the good points you hoped to stamp on the progeny become fixed but also some of the faults. This is often the case when the matings are arranged more on the basis of studying the pedigrees than the two dogs themselves to be mated in this way. No dog with any bad feature at all should be mated with another bearing the same feature.

In-breeding fixes characteristics, and with sensible selection very superior progeny can be produced, though very often this improvement is only noted in one or two of the litter. In-breeding is not a hundred per cent method of getting what you want in all the puppies, very far from it, but it is the shortest known cut to stamping a family likeness on the litters you breed. Unfortunately it often leads to a deterioration of constitution, size and temperament, and what you gain upon the swings you may lose upon the roundabouts. In-breeding is not an unnatural phenomenon. Formerly when dogs ran wild in packs the most powerful male was the sire of all the puppies in the pack and that of course led to intensive in-breeding. But what we are inclined to forget is that in those days the survival of the fittest was the rule, and the weaklings never survived. In these days of specialised dog-breeding when puppies mean money, even the weakest in the litter may be hand-reared, which is, of course, a very bad thing for the race.

Not all in-breeding is harmful, or sure to make the strain lose vigour, or produce bad temperament. These faults occur also with matings between completely unrelated animals, and one is far more likely to know what one is going to get as the result of in-breeding than by indiscriminate breeding from an unknown, unrelated sire. If the same constitutional weakness appears in both sides of the parents to be in-bred, then undoubtedly that weakness will be stamped in a terrifying way on the progeny. If, however, the breeder remembers to in-breed sensibly by only choosing vigorous fertile parents, rejecting all signs of any weakness, the resulting puppies should have indelibly stamped in them the good qualities sought after. I do not feel it is wise for amateur breeders to indulge in this method of breeding. It entirely depends on the skill used by the selector of the dogs to be mated.

Line-breeding is an entirely different process, and some of the best dogs in the world owe their beauty, temperament and vigour to being line-bred for generations. This is of course done chiefly on pedigree as well as selection, but you do not stamp the particular quality you require so quickly on the progeny as you do with in-breeding.

THE MATING

Having chosen your male sire for the future litter by pedigree, by seeing his offspring, and by noting the qualities you wish impressed on the offspring – above all his masculinity and temperament – you will have the job of seeing if your bitch likes the chosen mate. The bitch stays on heat anything up to twenty-one days, but for the first seven days she is passing a blood-stained discharge and will not allow male dogs near her. After the discharge ceases, she will usually be ready to mate on about the ninth to the fifteenth day, but there are variations on either side of these dates.

Unfortunately some bitches are distinctly shy breeders and absolutely refuse to have anything to do with the dog chosen for them. This can be extremely annoying. Nowadays artificial insemination is being used in rare cases and no doubt in the future will be used more and more, but unless such facilities are available, natural mating is still essential, and if the bitch is determined to have nothing to do with the dog of the owner's choice, she may have to be allowed the last word in the matter of choosing a sire. One golden rule to observe is never to breed with a bitch in her first season, but wait, until she comes into season for a second time. This will give her the necessary time to mature, and therefore her chances of conceiving will be greatly enhanced.

One can sometimes hold the bitch in position for the dog if she is really ready to be mated, which one can test by taking her near the dog when she will stand provocatively with her tail flat to her side, but I feel this is a bad thing and might cause injury to the bitch. Always let her play with the dog first, if possible somewhere where they can be alone but watched. She may at first be fickle and then suddenly decide to acquiesce. Sometimes difference of height makes mating difficult. Breeders use raised ground to counteract this or even a box like a seed box for a small dog to stand on. This mating of difficult cases should

really be left to experienced breeders; the average owner need only take her bitch along to the stud dog and call back for it. Some novices have been frightened at the length of time the dog and bitch are joined together, but remember this is a perfectly normal thing and calls for no interference.

Some people prefer to have the bitch mated twice, and of course, if the bitch were left with the dog they would mate many times, but this is not a good thing. For one thing you do not want too big a litter, especially for a young maiden bitch. Occasionally a terrible-looking puppy is born and the owner of the bitch runs to the owner of the stud dog and curses her, but it may simply be a throw-back or 'atavism' as it is called, and nobody can tell which side has this hereditary tendency. In such cases it is wiser not to use the same stud dog again. If the same thing happens again with a litter fathered by another sire it means, of course, that it is due to the bitch, and she is not one to use for breeding purposes. In cases where a mating does not induce pregnancy, the usual thing is for the bitch to be entitled to one free re-mating.

STERILITY

This can be due to a number of things. Lack of 'oestrus', or heat as it is known, is a common cause. Bitches usually come on heat for the first time between the ages of six and nine months and this is most commonly in spring and autumn, but nowadays under artificial conditions bitches show oestrus at any time of the year. Then again twice annually is the usual thing, but some of the small breeds only come on heat once a year. Sterility can be caused by the absence of ova, or by stunted growth which affects the genital organs. It may also be due to nymphomania, which causes the bitch to be almost continually on heat and which is in most cases due to chronic inflammation of the ovary; sometimes it is even caused by cysts. Only an examination by a vet can help in these cases. The lack of vitamin E has been found to cause sterility, as has, to some extent, excessive fat. Too much in-breeding causes weakness of the strain and is a contributory factor to sterility.

A lot of sterility is caused by the male dog; the absence of sperms, a deficiency of semen, and excess fat are all causes, and examination of the semen under a microscope will determine if lack of live spermatozoa is the cause. Naturally any disease in either male or female may also result in temporary, if not permanent, sterility. Nowadays the judicious use of hormone products helps to reduce sterility.

BITCHES IN WHELP

At the time of mating the egg cells or ova as they are called leave the bitch's ovary and find their way into the Fallopian tube. The male spermatozoa move up through the womb, or uterus as it is called, into the Fallopian tube where they fuse with the female ova. These then start to divide and after a few days reach the uterus where they burrow into the thickened lining membrane. They go on dividing and form the chorion or caul, as it is commonly known by most people. This protects the puppies during pregnancy and also nourishes them. This nourishing part is known as the placenta; here the interchange of food, oxygen and waste products occurs between puppies and their dam. But the two blood systems are divided by a thin membrane so that the mother and her puppies have separate blood supplies. Meanwhile the cells of the ova are developing into the puppies you will eventually know.

I will give you roughly the rate of growth of the foetus:

At ten days the ova are approximately one-twelfth to one-twentieth of an inch long.

At three to four weeks old they are approximately one inch in length.

At six weeks old they are approximately three inches long.

At seven to eight weeks old they are approximately five inches long. At the ninth week they are six to eight inches long.

The stages of development are interesting as well.

At ten days the fertilised ova have reached uterus.

At ten to twenty-one days traces of the foetus appear and traces of head, body and limbs can be discerned.

At three to four weeks the first indications of claws can be seen. At the fifth week the stomach is well defined.

At six weeks large hairs appear on lips, eyelids, etc.

At seven to eight weeks the eyelashes have appeared and hair is beginning to appear at the tip of the tail, head, and extremities, and by the ninth week the puppy is getting fully covered with hair and ready for its birth.

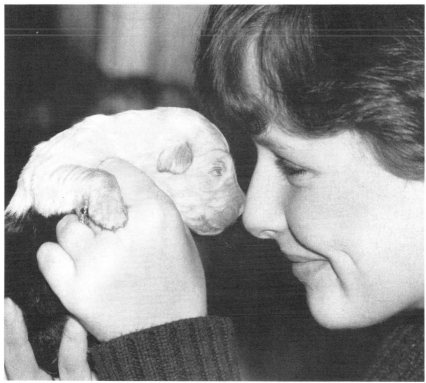

An Old English Sheepdog puppy – its eyes are now open.

The average bitch carries her litter for from fifty-eight to sixty-three days although it has been known for puppies to have been carried seventy days. Under fifty-eight days the puppies are unlikely to be alive. Milk should be a part of the bitch's diet and, if she likes it, occasionally fish and an egg. A varied diet at this time helps to provide all the vitamins necessary for healthy growth.

THE WHELPING

As whelping time approaches the bitch will become restless, she will have milk and will try and make a bed for herself. I have always found that if there is a nice warm cupboard in the kitchen or living-room bitches love to choose this for the birth of their litter. I usually put plenty of newspapers on the floor and then an old blanket. The puppies are each born separately in their foetal membranes but these should have ruptured as the puppy is born. If this does not happen they must be immediately ruptured by the owner; the afterbirth follows each birth. The navel string is usually bitten through by the mother; if this doesn't happen it must be cut. Normally, however, the owner need do nothing except watch the bitch to make sure she

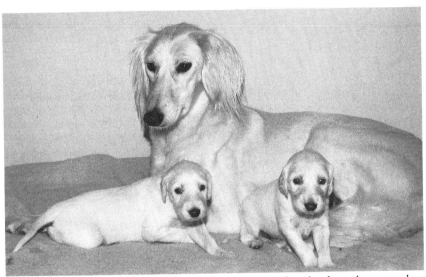

Most bitches will do everything for their puppies for the first three weeks.

doesn't savage her puppies. If she looks like doing this remove them as they are born and place them in a hot blanket kept warm by a hot bottle. Then return them to the mother after the last one is born. Make sure she has milk for them by squeezing the nipples and then leave her to suckle them in peace. When she has settled down, probably had a drink of warm milk and a little minced beef, you can change the soiled newspaper and blanket and make all clean and tidy.

The only time to really worry is if the bitch strains and strains and no puppy appears. If this is happening and the delay is unduly long between births it might mean a dead or deformed puppy and veterinary aid should be called. The other time to worry is if no births are occurring and a bloody or green discharge appears. Most owners suffer more than the bitch, and keep an eye on the clock wondering whether in fact they ought to call assistance. Only

experience will teach them, but most animals are best left to their own devices.

CARE OF THE LITTER

During the first three weeks the mother will do everything necessary for the care of the puppies. Incidentally, do not worry too much if she kicks one particular puppy out of the nest. Inexperienced owners keep putting it back, or even try rearing it on a bottle. I have always found if I have done this that there is something wrong with the puppy. The mother seems to know; therefore unless it is an extremely valuable one, I strongly advise that this one should be put down.

Start weaning the puppies at about three weeks old. Teach them to drink warm milk by putting a drop on the end of their muzzles; they will lick it off. Teach them to eat tiny morsels of

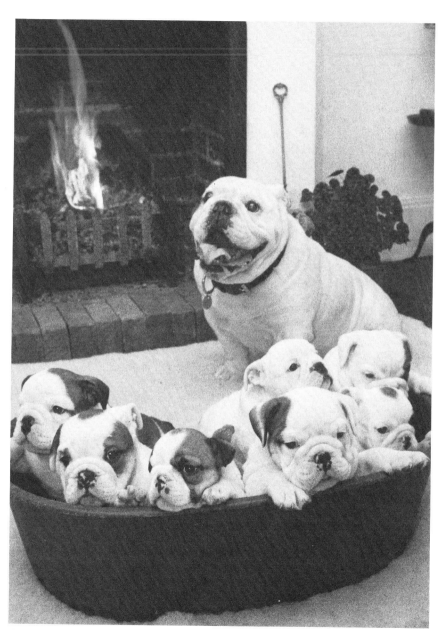

A nice evenly matched litter that has been well reared.

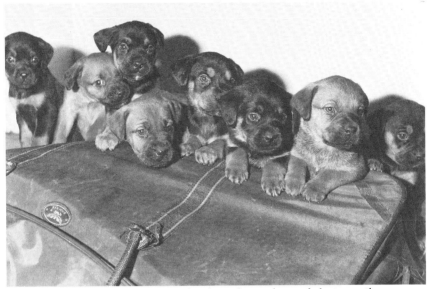

Soon the puppies will be completely independent of their mother.

minced beef by placing little pieces on the very tip of their tongues. In no time at all the puppies will be eager for this extra food and the bitch will move away from them quite a lot. By six weeks old they should be weaned, although some people like to give them another fortnight. They should in nice weather have been allowed to play in the sun on the lawn or a rug. That is why puppies born in the summer are so much easier to rear than winter-born puppies.

The puppies should be wormed at three months and again at six months; after that they should be all right. Puppies should have extra vitamins given to them, plenty of good food and fresh air, not forgetting warm, dry, and draught-proof sleeping quarters. They should never get over-tired by being mauled by children. It makes them irritable and they start to growl or snap at an early age. Handle them by all means but watch for the signal of the growl or wriggling away which shows they have had enough.

Teach them from the earliest days to be house clean; this is achieved by popping them out every two hours to the same spot with the same words 'Hurry up' and giving plenty of praise when they perform. A watchful owner seldom has a dirty puppy for long. Never teach them on newspaper, a filthy habit if ever there was one. If they must perform in a flat give them a tray of sand or turf. Association of ideas is everything, and no one wants a dog in later life to associate paper with relieving itself. Start how you mean to go on.

HAND REARING

In the vast majority of cases nature provides the mother with adequate milk to feed the number she produces. However there are, of course, cases where the milk supply of the dam is inadequate and the foster mother must be quickly found or hand-rearing resorted to, which is a terrible job. Every week in the dog papers such as *Dog World* and *Our Dogs* you will find advertisements of foster mothers. Sometimes your vet will know where a foster mother can be obtained. Sometimes a cat with newly-born kittens will suckle a puppy with great affection.

In any case if you hire a foster mother she will arrive with one of her own puppies as well and must be returned to her owner when the puppies are weaned. If the puppies are reared by hand, a patent bottle and teats can be bought at the chemist for this purpose. The bottles and teats must be kept scrupulously clean and the puppies fed every two hours day and night to begin with. There are a number of milk powder products on the market which are suitable for puppies.

Chapter Five

COMMON AILMENTS

WORM INFESTATION

There are numerous kinds of worms which infect dogs: intestinal, blood, stomach, among others – but the most common are the roundworms and tapeworms. Worms in puppies cause endless trouble and can be seen when passed as round white things pointed at both ends. The puppies are often pot-bellied, and if you look at the tummy it often has a bluish tinge. The coat is poor and the puppy often doesn't thrive. Contrarily I have seen puppies thrive very well who have, when wormed, passed large quantities of roundworms. They often have a terrific appetite, but the food does them no good. There are a mass of proprietary worm cures on the market. Personally I would recommend a beginner to send the puppy to the vet to be properly wormed, as they have stronger cures. Puppies should be wormed at twelve weeks and six months and then once more if any signs are seen.

People tend to say: "Where can my puppy have picked up worm?" The answer is, eating grass, drinking from pools, eating dung, and many other causes. Roundworms are not communicable to man but tapeworm is, and can cause a very serious disease of the muscles in man, so if any flat segments of worm are ever seen in the motions, the dog should be immediately treated for tapeworms. On no account whatsoever let the dog eat off plates or dishes used by human beings; do not kiss the dog, or let your face anywhere near his muzzle as they lick their rear portions and the eggs may be carried on the muzzle. These worms can cause paralysis in the dog. Rabbits are the intermediate host of tapeworms so it is dangerous to give raw rabbit, in my opinion. The dog should be treated professionally. Some puppies get worms through the blood stream of their dams: that is the reason the bitch should be wormed when pregnant in the early stages, or before mating. Cleanliness in everything to do with dogs is essential.

DIARRHOEA

Most dogs will suffer from this

periodically throughout their lives, and for most owners the worry is knowing whether it is caused by diet or disease. In fact, this is fairly simple. If the dog doesn't appear ill, has no temperature, and quickly responds to a change of diet and simple remedies you can be fairly sure that diet, or a slight chill, is the cause. But this looseness of the motion is an early symptom of so many diseases that if it persists more than one day you would be very wise to seek expert advice. Many dogs suffer an intolerance to fat and if their diet happens to contain too much they promptly get diarrhoea. They pass mucus and sometimes blood and the owner is terrified, but again the response to medication is usually prompt. A veterinary surgeon writes:

"Diarrhoea usually results from some irritation in the bowel during the course of an infectious disease or in cases of poisoning. It may commonly occur without other symptoms and may be the result of mild food-poisoning. Where vomiting occurs it is as well to withhold food for at least twenty-four hours, and only give water in regulated quantity, preferably with glucose. Again, with diarrhoea it is well to withhold food; glucose is useful and arrowroot and raw eggs will often help. It is impossible to suggest anything other than first-aid treatment before the cause of the condition is established."

SKIN DISEASES

Before discussing the management and treatment of dogs with skin diseases I feel the reader should know something about the structure of the hair. Practically the whole surface of the body of the dog is covered by hair. Even the stomach that looks so bare has very fine hairs, as you will see if you examine it closely. Dogs shed their coats twice a year but this is the major casting of the coat; actually hair is being shed all the time. That is one of the reasons that dogs should be groomed. There are many different types of hairs; for example, those big thick ones on the lips are called 'tactile' hairs, the eyelash hairs are called 'cilia', those that are found in the outer ear are termed 'tragi', and those found in the nostril 'vibrissae'. But to the ordinary dog owner they are just hairs. That part of the hair which can be seen above the surface of the skin is known as the 'shaft' and that below the skin is the 'bulb', capped by the expanded end of the hair root. The sebaceous glands, which produce an oily substance called 'sebum', open into the follicles of the hair a little way beneath the surface. It is these little glands which by their copious production make the coat shiny.

When certain skin diseases attack the dog the parasites enter the hair shaft or follicles and set up intense irritation. Mange is one of the most common of these and certain varieties are extremely contagious. It is caused by mange mites which look rather like tiny crabs and the Sarcoptes variety, which is the common one in dogs, has suckers on its legs. The treatment of all skin diseases, whether they are infectious or not, must start with a strict diet of health-giving food, with special attention to vitamins to keep the dog's strength up. Infectious mange must be treated professionally, and everything in contact with the dog should be destroyed. But there is one type of mange called 'follicular mange' which is common in Dachshunds, Boxers, Miniature Black-and-Tans, *etc.*, which is not infectious and which is believed to be passed on to the puppies by the mother before birth. At any rate, whether this is true or not, there certainly is a tendency for certain strains in these breeds and other short-coated similar types of dog to have this disease from a very early age. I once bought a miniature Black-and-Tan that had it at six weeks. The symptoms are bare patches under the necks and tummies; the tummies have little papular spots. Nowadays, although one does not knowingly buy a dog that comes from a strain so afflicted, the cure is easy, namely washing the dog with Tetmosol soap and leaving the soap in.

Eczema, however, is an entirely different type of trouble. It has been proved that its cause is largely dietetic and several people have evolved a natural diet that seems to work wonders in these cases. But besides being dietetic in cause I believe this is a nervous disease akin to asthma in humans, and if ordinary diet changes fail to cure it, I suggest the proteins in the food be changed until the element to which the dog is allergic is eliminated, when the condition should clear up. Allergic conditions of this sort have been found to respond magically to certain antihystamine preparations, which I think proves that dogs, as well as humans, suffer from allergies. Calamine lotion applied to the raw patches relieves the irritation as well. The main thing is to prevent the dog biting and scratching himself; this is done by enveloping his paws in boots and making him wear a large flat leather collar which prevents him reaching

himself on his body to bite it. Most vets have such collars. It is always better to take expert advice to find out what your dog is suffering from before attempting home treatment, though, as a general rule, fat should certainly be cut out of the diet and greenstuffs added.

TRAVEL SICKNESS

Dogs are usually sick in cars because they are looking out of the sides of the car rather than the front. They are sick because they are nervous and don't really trust their owners. The only way to get over this is to train them thoroughly in obedience so that they lie down and stay down quietly in the car; then they will not be sick. I once took a drive with a Red Setter bitch that had never been driven in a car without being sick in the first few minutes. I sat in the back with her and ordered her to lie down, in my firmest tone. Incidentally she was a pupil in my training school and knew that when I gave a command I meant it to be obeyed. She lay down, head on my lap, and never showed the slightest sign of being sick or even dribbling. This, in my opinion, supports my theory that the owner is to blame for not giving confidence to the dog.

I think it wrong to feed a dog before a journey. Water should be available and reasonable exercise at not too long intervals. I think sedatives can be extremely useful if a long journey is contemplated, because the owner will be worrying as to whether the dog is going to be sick and it will pick up her fears and probably be sick. It might even be more effective if the owner took the sedative!

Always have a puppy's head on your

lap when teaching it to be happy in a car. If the puppy is on the floor the vibrations and the smell from the car will make him sick. As everyone knows with children, fresh air helps to overcome sickness. Dogs, however, should not be allowed to put their heads out of the window for fear of injuring their eyes. Take your dogs constantly with you everywhere from the time they first come to you and you will have no trouble. I am positive car sickness is an allergy to cars and the surroundings.

Chapter Six

FIRST AID

I think every household with a dog in it should have a first-aid box, clearly labelled with the contents, and possibly a list of what to do in an emergency. It is extraordinary how many people panic when something has happened to their dog. My own first-aid box contains, among other things: bicarbonate of soda for application to bee stings and an application for wasp stings. Milton is invaluable; it should be kept in every first-aid box for antiseptic treatment of cuts and burns, and is also extremely useful for sterilising utensils when there is a sick dog in the house.

CUTS

I will deal first with cuts. These can be little more than scratches or they can be deep cuts which need expert attention. The way to tell whether a severe cut has severed an artery or not is by watching how the blood comes. If it comes in a pumping fashion in time with the pulse, there is severance of the artery and bleeding must be stopped at all costs or you may lose your dog. The best method if bleeding is severe is to apply

a tourniquet above the wound. This is done by wrapping a clean handkerchief round the limb, if the injury is in a leg or paw, and putting a pencil into the handkerchief and twisting until the bleeding stops. The pressure should be applied above the wound and on the side of the injury nearest the heart. It is important not to have the tourniquet too tight so that it harms the limb, but just tight enough to stop the bleeding. It should be loosened every ten minutes or so to see if the bleeding is arrested.

If the bleeding comes from a vein, in which case the flow of blood will be regular, the tourniquet should be applied below the injury. If this is not possible, apply pressure over a pad directly on the wound. The blood from an artery is always brighter than that from a vein. The dog should have veterinary aid as soon as possible, and any deep or very ragged wound is best stitched by a vet. It is not often that such bad injuries occur in dogs except when injured on the road or cut by wire or glass. But dogs do often receive minor scratches and cuts, and if these are washed with 10 volume peroxide or a solution of Milton and kept clean afterwards, they heal very rapidly.

Normally wounds heal by what we term 'granulating inwards'. Granulations are small masses of cells containing loops of freshly formed blood-vessels which form on the healing surface of the wound and in multiplying, close in the wound until the whole surface is healed over. Occasionally this process gets out of hand and excessive granulation takes place and this is known as 'proud flesh'. The wound will not heal with proud flesh, and that part above the surface of the wound must be burnt back with a silver nitrate stick, when normal healing will occur. Dogs are particularly bad at keeping wounds open by licking them, so where the wound can have a stitch it has more likelihood of healing quickly. I loathe iodine for first aid. It can be extremely dangerous owing to its tendency to seal the wound and shut the germs in. Also some dogs are sensitive to iodine and the reaction is worse than the wound.

BRUISES

A bruise is a contusion where the skin is not broken. The bleeding occurs under the skin, hence the discoloration of the tissues. Bruises need cold-water bandages or the hose gently running over them. I have found homeopathic tincture of calendula makes an excellent cold compress diluted with water and applied on a pad to the bruise. I used it extensively in Argentina for humans and animals when they got hurt. It can be bought from any chemist who stocks homeopathic remedies.

GRASS SEEDS

Occasionally dogs get grass seeds in their eyes and are in terrible pain. The first-aid treatment is castor oil in the eye as quickly as possible, and then take the dog to the vet. He will know if serious damage has been done by staining the eye with fluorescence, which remains in the scratch but washes off the normal uninjured surface. Should there be a scratch on the cornea, cortisone drops are usually instilled into the eye and healing takes place. It is essential to stop the dog rubbing the injured eye. Sometimes grass seeds enter the ear and cause a lot of trouble. Once again, beyond putting a little warm oil into the ear, you can do nothing; it is an expert's job because with an auriscope, which looks rather like a torch, the vet can look right into the ear and remove the offending grass seed.

BURNS

Burns and scalds have been known to occur when the household dog has bumped into the busy housewife and caused her to spill boiling water over him. The first-aid treatment is to cut off the hair and apply moist bicarbonate of soda to the affected part. Should it be a third-degree burn with a blister, don't break the blister. Cover it up with bicarbonate of soda and place a damp clean rag over it. Get qualified aid quickly. In all cases of severe injury the dog is probably suffering from shock and should be kept warm by a fire or with a blanket over him. If he will drink some warm milk, that helps to combat shock.

FRACTURES

If you suspect a fracture, do not move the dog. Apply a splint and bandage lightly. It is important to get the dog to the vet as quickly as possible so that it can be X-rayed. With careful nursing, there is no reason why the dog should not be able to make a complete recovery from this injury.

CHOKING

Choking is sometimes experienced by dogs, and it is very frightening for the owner. If a piece of bone is choking the dog you should try and dislodge it by crooking your little finger and making an effort to bring the offending piece of bone back. Bones, unless they are unbroken shinbones, should never be given to dogs, in my opinion.

Chapter Seven

CANINE CONDITIONS

I feel the nursing of animals is very similar to the nursing of human beings. The place where they are nursed should be kept warm yet airy. The carpet should be protected or removed if the dog has bowel or kidney trouble or is likely to be sick. A coal fire, if this is possible, is the best method of heating the room as it provides not only heat but ventilation as well. Ample water should always be available unless the vet for any specific reason has forbidden this. A cottonwool coat should be made for the dog if he has pneumonia and provision for changing his bedding should also be made.

The diet should be attractive to the dog, but remember that the patient is not taking his usual exercise; to overfeed him or press him to take something he doesn't want can only be injurious. Whites of egg slip easily down the dog's throat via the loose lips and the natural pouch of the dog's cheek, and dogs can live on this diet alone for some time. Meat tea made from beef or veal can be jellied and easily administered to the dog. I have found that rabbit's liver will be eaten when

everything else has failed to tempt. Brains, and of course milk, are excellent for the sick dog. Anything that is concentrated and easily digested can keep the dog's strength up and nourish the body without unduly taxing the digestive organs. If the dog takes something voluntarily it is worth much more than forcing food down him, and he is less likely to regurgitate it.

One thing that may make my readers smile is my advice not to sympathize with your dog too much when ill. If I say to my dog 'Poor Juno! you do look ill', she wilts visibly until she really does look ill. The power of mind over matter counts with dogs as well as with human beings. To leave the dog to sleep or rest as much as possible is another important part of nursing. Naturally one is so very anxious that one is inclined to return constantly to the dog hoping for signs of improvement, but these disturbances retard the dog's progress as often as not. Peace and quiet, cleanliness in every matter connected with the patient, warmth with adequate draught-free ventilation are the general rules for the nursing of a sick dog.

ABCESSES

Abscesses can be caused purely and simply by bacteria and, of course, the cure then is to administer antibiotics. Occasionally, though, abscesses are subcutaneous ones, not filled with pus but with blood serum, and that type clears up pretty quickly on opening. If the abscess is a pus-filled one, fomenting frequently with hot water until the head has turned yellow is the best treatment. The abscess can then be punctured and the pus let out and an antibiotic cream like aureomycin or penicillin placed on a piece of clean linen over the wound. Keep the wound open until all infection has subsided.

ARTHRITIS

Whilst arthritis is a fairly specific sort of word actually meaning an inflammation of a joint, rheumatism is one of those rather vague terms which is loosely used to cover a multitude of conditions mainly causing pain on movement or pressure. The cause of this seems to be somewhat obscure, but it is certain that dogs are commonly affected by a condition causing muscular pain, which is aggravated by movement. It is most commonly seen in older animals and frequently occurs when exercise is irregular. It is sometimes seen, for instance, in working dogs when they have a very long day which has been preceded by several days rest. It is also frequently seen when the animal has become wet and chilled and it may affect many different groups of muscles.

It is probably most common in the muscles of the back, the shoulders and the jaw, but it may be difficult to localise as almost any movement may cause distant muscles to contract. Warmth, rest and aspirin seem to be the best first-aid methods when this type of condition is suspected. A mild laxative should also be given as animals frequently find it difficult to assume the position for defecation. It is impossible to define the symptoms of arthritis because almost any joint in the body may be affected. There is usually some degree of heat and pain over the affected area, as well as lameness, if a leg is involved. Sometimes arthritis can be a very slowly developing condition and is difficult to diagnose without the use of X-ray. It is often seen when any form of wound actually penetrates the joint capsule.

The joints of the spine are particularly complex in that the vertebrae are all separated by pads, which are usually referred to as discs. Occasionally, due to injury or to age, or more commonly to the necessary predisposition in the long-backed dog, portions of these discs protrude and in this case they usually interfere with the functioning of the nerves leading from the spine, and some degree of paralysis varying from a slight staggering gait to a complete paralysis follows. This condition is frequently very painful in the early stages. Treatment of these cases is rather prolonged and considerable nursing skill may be required to assist dogs in emptying their bowels and their bladders. Professional advice should be sought and often X-ray examination is necessary to clarify diagnosis.

CYSTS, INTERDIGITAL

There are many different opinions as to

what causes these interdigital cysts. I think most people agree that somehow organisms have entered the tissues where these suppurating swellings appear, and caused hard painful lumps which the dogs lick and lick. They burst and heal up and then, very often, break out again. They often clear up after incision and treatment with some antibiotic. With my own dog aureomycin has worked like magic, but most vets have their own ideas on the best treatment for each individual case. Hot fomentations are extremely good and can very often save an incision.

Dogs that get out of condition are more likely to get these cysts, and I have found a course of vitamins an enormous help in preventing their appearance. I am positive walking on newly-tarred or concrete surfaces is a major cause of trouble, and I do not think grass seeds a likely explanation.

CYSTITIS

Cystitis or inflammation of the bladder affects bitches and is usually caused by a chill. The bitch will cry out when her bladder is pressed and may also cry out when she passes urine. This trouble is usually quickly knocked out by antibiotics. This complaint is not to be mixed up with cysts or tumours.

DIABETES

If you suspect your dog has diabetes the first thing to do is to have his urine tested for sugar. Diabetes is a condition in which an excess of grape sugar is found in the urine due to a deficiency of the internal secretion of the pancreas. When a synthetic preparation is made

from the islet cells of the pancreas and is injected in the correct quantities into the body this excess sugar disappears from the urine. Sometimes diabetes leads also to a cataract which affects the eyesight, and the dog becomes very sluggish. In my opinion it is kinder to put a dog to sleep if he develops diabetes, as continually repeated injections are the only treatment, and to give these is not very kind to the animal.

ENTROPION

This condition is caused by inverted eyelids; some say it is hereditary, others believe that it is caused by inflammation of the conjunctiva or lining of the lids. The cure is to take away by surgery an elliptical piece of skin from the outer surface of the eyelid and stitch the edges together again, which causes the lashes to turn outwards once more. The dog suffers very little discomfort. The opposite sort of thing sometimes happens in dogs, and that is the turning outwards of the conjunctiva or lining of the eyelid, and then the operation is to remove part of the conjunctiva from the inside of the lid. This condition is normal in dogs like Bloodhound and St Bernard, but can look very nasty in other dogs.

While we are on the subject of eyes I should mention that dogs sometimes get warts on their eyelids. They spread at an alarming rate and, in my opinion, you should seek expert veterinary advice immediately they are noticed or blindness may ensue. Inflammation of the eyelids is termed blepharitis and can be extremely dangerous and cause blindness, although in these days of cortisone and other drugs, better treatment can be hoped for. It is not a disease that should be treated at home, and I strongly advise you to consult your vet without delay. It may be a simple condition caused by dust or hay seed or it may not. The dog will probably have an intolerance to light if it is blepharitis, so keep him in a darkened room until the vet comes.

HEATSTROKE

Excessive panting may indicate distress and dogs should be taken into a shady or cool place or they may get a heatstroke. It is not unknown for dogs to die at shows in hot weather through having heatstroke. If a stroke is threatened immediately put cold compresses to the head, or if the temperature is extremely high immerse the dog in cold water until the temperature is reduced to about 103 degrees Fahrenheit, which is fairly safe for a dog. Of course the animal must be dried off or chill may result. Cool drinks where the animal is conscious are invaluable. Shutting dogs in cars with the windows closed is one cause of heatstroke. Only thoughtless owners would do such a thing.

KIDNEY TROUBLE

If you were to read about kidneys in a veterinary book, you would probably become very little the wiser. It is quite a complex subject. Roughly speaking, however, the kidneys are in the body to excrete urine and to act as selective filters allowing only the passage of the water and salts and keeping back albumen and sugar. If the dog eats something like mouldy dog biscuits this may set up congestion of the kidneys, and the kidneys have to work overtime passing urine trying to relieve the congestion. This congestion can be caused by a bacterial infection, but the resulting excessive passage of urine is nearly the same. Antibiotics form part of the treatment. Warmth, laxative, easily digested food, and barley water all give the kidneys the rest they need to return to normal. Kidney trouble should never be taken lightly and professional advice should be sought early. It is because it is so important that I have asked a vet to write on this subject at some length:

"Several diseases of an infectious nature affect primarily the liver or the kidneys of the dog:

INFECTIOUS VIRAL HEPATITIS (Rhubarth' s disease)

Although this condition is caused by a virus it does not seem to be as readily infectious, even in kennels, as one might expect. This may possibly be because some dogs are infected but the disease in them is so mild that it passes unnoticed. Other animals may show almost any signs from a slight passing illness to the acute disease with death in a few hours or days. In the mild form diagnosis is extremely difficult, but in the more acute types the animal becomes very depressed, has a rise in temperature, increasing thirst, vomiting and pain in the forward part of the floor of the abdomen. Food is usually refused and diarrhoea may occur; the vomit is usually yellow and bile-stained and the animal becomes increasingly dehydrated. In the most acute forms so much damage is done to the liver that death occurs rapidly.

LEPTOSPIROSIS

There are two types of this disease. The first is caused by the organism called Leptospira icterohcmorrhagica, most commonly called "jaundice" or "the yellows". This germ primarily affects the liver and the inflammation in that organ prevents the natural release of bile. It is bile circulating in the blood which causes the yellow discoloration which is such a marked symptom in the later stages of the disease. The animal loses its appetite, becomes very depressed and frequently runs a high temperature. Vomiting is fairly frequent, at first white, then yellow. After a while yellow discoloration begins to appear and is most noticeable in the white of the eye and the gums. In light-coloured dogs the skin of the abdomen is also noticeably yellow. All food is refused and there is usually an increased thirst, the animal vomiting up everything it drinks within a few moments. Depression is marked, dehydration occurs rapidly and is followed by death, in extreme cases, five or six days after the onset of symptoms.

"The trained observer will notice that the membranes of the eyes and mouth become dark and congested before the yellow discoloration appears. Treatment in these cases again consists of good nursing. Warmth and repeated small doses of fluids, preferably with glucose, are essential. A serum is available and antibiotics (penicillin, streptomycin, etc.) are also of value. A preventative vaccine is also available and may be used any time after four months of age. This particular germ affects many different animals including, occasionally, man, and the common rat is the usual cause

of spread. The germs are excreted in the saliva and the urine.

"The second is Leptospira canicola. This germ is closely related to the one causing jaundice, but it usually causes an inflammation of the kidneys (Nephritis) of varying severity. It is known that very many dogs are infected, often without showing signs of illness but leaving the kidneys affected, which is probably the reason why chronic nephritis is one of the commonest causes of death in the older male dog. Frequently, however, the disease causes varying degrees of illness. The symptoms may vary considerably, but there is usually a rise in temperature and a loss of appetite, vomiting and diarrhoea. Pain is usually present in the kidney region and membranes may become congested at first, and later, rather pale with, sometimes, very small haemorrhages on the gums. The breath becomes very unpleasant and the teeth sometimes stained. A very good percentage of cases recover if professional help is sought in time."

PARAPHIMOSIS

This occurs more in small dogs than large ones. It is caused by the orifice of the sheath being rather small and contracting on the penis when this has protruded; the latter then becomes swollen and painful and cannot be retracted without help. If not noticed early the point of the penis becomes much inflamed. The treatment should be to try and ease the sheath over the penis again, if necessary putting a little medicinal paraffin oil on the penis to lubricate it. If the dog will allow it, ice helps to reduce the swelling. The dog should be lying on its back or side to carry out this treatment. If all first aid fails, the vet may have to make a snip in the prepuce to allow the penis to retract.

PNEUMONIA

Nowadays antibiotics have made pneumonia a far less dangerous condition than it was. It is not common in dogs, usually occurring only as a complication to some other disease like hard-pad or distemper. But it can be a secondary infection after an accident, or even just a common cold, if the dog is allowed to get chilled or wet. The symptoms are shivering with a rising temperature, which may reach 104 degrees Fahrenheit or even more. The respirations are rapid and painful, and if you have any experience of these things place your ear against the dog's ribs behind the front leg where you will hear a grating inspiration and expiration. It takes experience to recognise these sounds, though, and in any case the owner of a dog affected by pneumonia would be well advised to get professional advice. In pneumonia the dog usually stays lying on his side.

The first thing to do is to make the dog a pneumonia jacket and you can buy gauze-covered cotton wool for this from any chemist. It requires a hole for the head and front paws and then tapes sewn on to keep it in place. The whole treatment of pneumonia depends on the use of antibiotics and on keeping the dog warm while allowing him fresh air to help his breathing. The dog's appetite is bad, therefore light nourishing food should be given. The bowels should be kept in a laxative state, and this can be assisted by giving a purge at first and then liquid medicinal paraffin. The drugs needed for the treatment of pneumonia cannot be obtained by the ordinary owner; it is essential to employ a vet to handle the case as soon as possible.

TONSILITIS

If a dog's tonsils and throat are red, that definitely points to tonsilitis. As a sore throat can be the start of many diseases, it is wise to take the dog's temperature and consult your vet. First-aid treatment is, of course, just like that of a human being: a half to a whole aspirin according to size, and keep the patient warm. This is where antibiotics come to the rescue if it is anything more than a mild case. The dog should be given soft foods like minced beef, milk, and a little honey if he will take it.

TUMOURS

Malignant tumours or cancer, the name by which they are better known, occurs when there is a sudden multiplying of certain cells of the tissues and the eating through of the bone. If the malignant tumour does not involve bone substance, as for example in cancer of the mammary tissue, an operation in the early stages can be most effective, however, in many cases the tumour grows so rapidly that the prognosis is poor. Consult your vet immediately when you find an unknown swelling, wherever it may be; it may only be a cyst, in which case it can easily be removed.

APPENDIX

A range of other books, tapes and accessories are available to help you derive the full benefit from the Barbara Woodhouse approach to dog training.

Other titles in this series are:

Barbara Woodhouse On How Your Dog Thinks

Barbara looks at the world from the dog's viewpoint, and comes up with some new and surprising theories on dog behaviour. She shows owners how to understand their dogs and to communicate with them, not just by words and commands, but by tone of voice, and body language. In this book Barbara Woodhouse uses her rare gifts to break down the barriers, and helps all owners to achieve perfect companionship with their dogs.

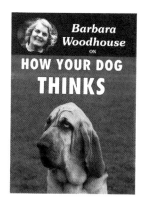

Barbara Woodhouse On Training Your Dog

Barbara guides the owner through the first steps of basic obedience, essential for the family pet, and graduates, stage by stage, to more advanced and specialised training. This book is essential for every owner who wants their dog to be "a pleasure to all, and a nuisance to none."

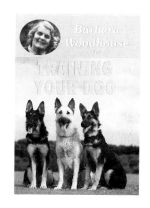

Barbara Woodhouse On Handling A Problem Dog

Whether it is an aggressive dog, a nervous dog, a roaming dog or a thief, Barbara Woodhouse believes that with proper understanding, most faults can be cured quickly and a happy relationship can be built up between owner and dog. At this time, more than any other, it is essential that all dogs are well behaved and live in harmony with their owners and with society. Barbara, who has trained some 19,000 dogs, tackles a wide spectrum of 'problem dogs' and comes up with sound, commonsense solutions.

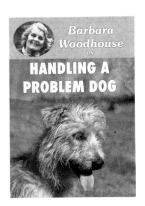

Barbara Woodhouse On How To Train Your Puppy

Barbara gives invaluable advice on house training, diet, exercise, and early training, and perhaps most important of all, she helps new owners get off to the right start, so that they can achieve a happy working relationship with their dog.

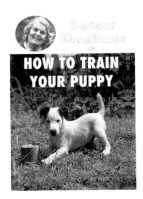

All these titles should be available through your local pet or book shop, price £3.99 each. In cases of difficulty they can be ordered direct from the publisher.
(Please add 75p per title towards P&P).
See address at the end of this section.

60

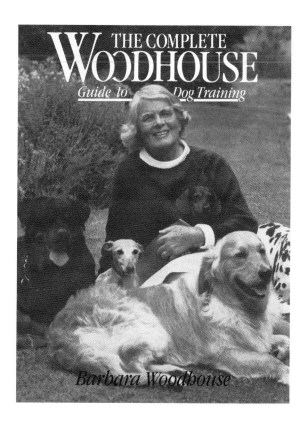

The Complete Woodhouse Guide To Dog Training

This is the definitive volume on dog training from Britain's best-loved expert.
Everything you need to know about the care and control of your dog; how to
understand his behaviour and how to get the best from him.
This book contains the very best of Barbara Woodhouse's writing
on a subject she understands like no other.
Available from good bookshops everywhere, price £14.95

*In case of difficulty The Complete Woodhouse Guide To Dog Training
can be ordered direct from the publisher.*
***(Please add £1.50 towards P&P).
See address at the end of this section.***

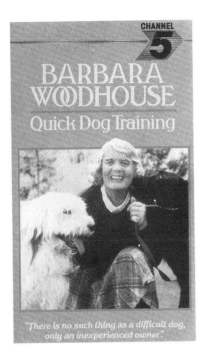

And if you've read the book, it is time to see the movie!

THE *WOODHOUSE* VIDEO
Barbara Woodhouse:
Quick Dog Training

A complete programme of obedience exercises for you and your dog. This 90 minute video takes you step-by-step through all the essential commands: Sit, Stay, Wait, Down, Leave and Recall. *PLUS* house training, giving medicine, obedience in the car and on the street, walking to heel and much, much more from the most celebrated dog trainer in the world.

Price: £14.99
(plus £1.50 P&P)

Available ONLY from the publisher.
See address at the end of this section

BARBARA WOODHOUSE
CHOKE CHAINS AND LEADS
Are also available through the publisher

CHOKE CHAINS

Sizes at two–inch intervals
Twelve inches to eighteen inches   £3.00
Twenty inches to Twenty-eight inches   £3.50

To obtain the correct choke chain, measure over the top of the dog's
head, down over the ears and under the chin, then add two inches
and round up or down to the nearest size.
Please add 95p P&P to each order

LEADS

Approx four foot long in best quality bridle leather
Large or small trigger hooks   £5.95
Please add 95p P&P to each order

BARBARA WOODHOUSE AUDIO CASSETTE

BASED ON THE SERIES
TRAINING DOGS THE WOODHOUSE WAY
Price: £5.95
(including postage and packing)

HOW TO ORDER

All the items described here can be ordered
direct from the publisher

RINGPRESS BOOKS LTD.,
SPIRELLA HOUSE, BRIDGE ROAD,
LETCHWORTH, HERTS SG6 4ET

Please remember to add postage and packing charge where
necessary and allow 21 days for delivery.

ACCESS and VISA card holder may order by telephone on
0462 674177

Office open 9am to 5pm Monday to Friday